RENAL DIET RECIPES 2021

-Quick and Delicious Recipes with Low Quantities of Potassium, Sodium and Phosphorus for Every Stage of Kidney Disease-

[Simona Malcom]

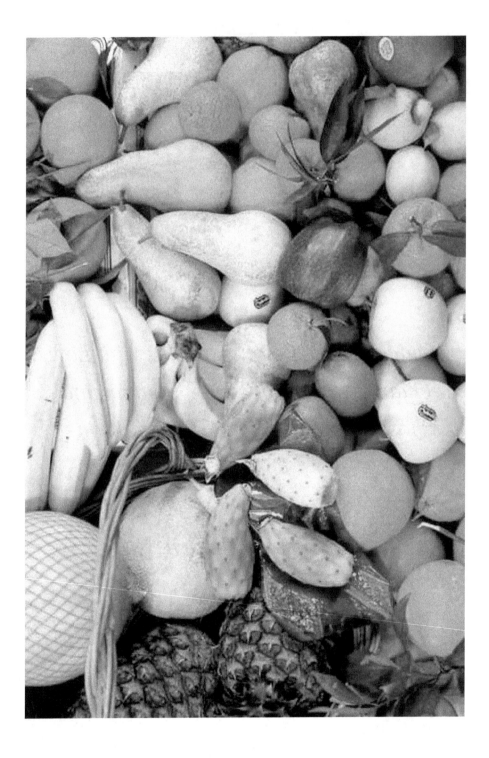

Table Of Contents

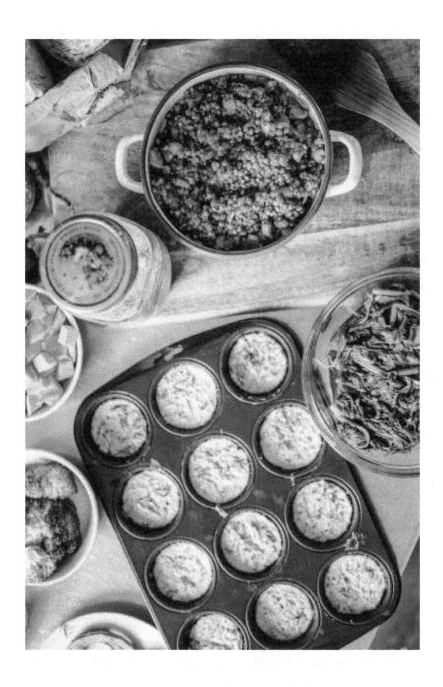

The following Book is reproduced below with the goal of providing information that is as accurate and reliable as possible. Regardless, purchasing this Book can be seen as consent to the fact that both the publisher and the author of this book are in no way experts on the topics discussed within and that any recommendations or suggestions that are made herein are for entertainment purposes only. Professionals should be consulted as needed prior to undertaking any of the action endorsed herein.

This declaration is deemed fair and valid by both the American Bar Association and the Committee of Publishers Association and is legally binding throughout the United States.

Furthermore, the transmission, duplication, or reproduction of any of the following work including specific information will be considered an illegal act irrespective of if it is done electronically or in print. This extends to creating a secondary or tertiary copy of the work or a recorded copy and is only allowed with the express written consent from the Publisher. All additional right reserved.

The information in the following pages is broadly considered a truthful and accurate account of facts and as such, any inattention, use, or misuse of the information in question by the reader will render any resulting actions solely under their purview. There are no scenarios in which the publisher or the original author of this work can be in any fashion deemed liable for any hardship or damages that may befall them after undertaking information described herein.

Additionally, the information in the following pages is intended only for informational purposes and should thus be thought of as universal. As befitting its nature, it is presented without assurance regarding its prolonged validity or interim quality. Trademarks that are mentioned are done without written consent and can in no way be considered an endorsement from the trademark holder.

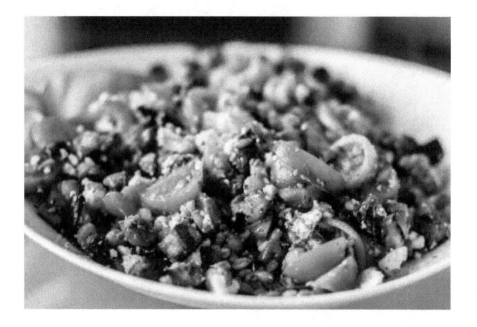

Introduction

Human health hangs in a complete balance when all of its interconnected bodily mechanisms function properly in perfect sync. Without its major organs working normally, the body soon suffers indelible damage. Kidney malfunction is one such example, and it is not just the entire water balance that is disturbed by the kidney disease, but a number of other diseases also emerge due to this problem.

Kidney diseases are progressive, meaning that they can ultimately lead to permanent kidney damage if left unchecked and uncontrolled. That is why it is essential to control and manage the disease and halt its progress, which can be done through medicinal and natural means. While medicines can guarantee only thirty percent of the cure, a change of lifestyle and diet can prove miraculous with their seventy percent guaranteed results. A kidney-friendly diet and lifestyle not only saves the kidneys from excess minerals, but it also aids medicines to work actively. Treatment without a good diet, hence, proves to be useless. In this renal diet cookbook, we shall bring out the basic facts about kidney diseases, their symptoms, causes, and diagnosis. This preliminary introduction can help the readers understand the problem clearly; then, we shall discuss the role of renal diet and kidney-friendly lifestyle in curbing the diseases. It's not just that the book also contains a range of delicious renal diet recipes, which will guarantee luscious flavors and good health.

Despite their tiny size, the kidneys perform a number of functions, which are vital for the body to be able to function healthily.

These include:

- Filtering excess fluids and waste from the blood.

- Creating the enzyme known as renin, which regulates blood pressure.

- Ensuring bone marrow creates red blood cells.

- Controlling calcium and phosphorus levels through absorption and excretion.

Unfortunately, when kidney disease reaches a chronic stage, these functions start to stop working. However, with the right treatment and lifestyle, it is possible to manage symptoms and continue living well. This is even more applicable in the earlier stages of the disease. Tactlessly, 10% of all adults over the age of 20 will experience some form of kidney disease in their lifetime. There are a variety of different treatments for kidney disease, which depend on the cause of the disease.

According to international stats, kidney (or renal) diseases are affecting around 14% of the adult population. In the US, approx. 661.000 Americans suffer from kidney dysfunction. Out of these patients, 468.000 proceed to dialysis treatment, and the rest have one active kidney transplant.

The high quantities of diabetes and heart illness are also related to kidney dysfunction, and sometimes one condition, for example, diabetes, may prompt the other.

With such a significant number of high rates, possibly the best course of treatment is the contravention of dialysis, making people depend upon clinical and crisis facility meds in any occasion multiple times every week. In this manner, if your kidney has just given a few indications of brokenness, you can forestall dialysis through an eating routine, something that we will talk about in this book.

CHAPTER 1: The Renal Diet

The Benefits of Renal diet

If you have been diagnosed with kidney dysfunction, a proper diet is necessary for controlling the amount of toxic waste in the bloodstream. When toxic waste piles up in the system along with increased fluid, chronic inflammation occurs, and we have a much higher chance of developing cardiovascular, bone, metabolic, or other health issues.

Since your kidneys can't fully get rid of the waste on their own, which comes from food and drinks, probably the only natural way to help our system is through this diet.

A renal diet is especially useful during the first stages of kidney dysfunction and leads to the following benefits:

● Prevents excess fluid and waste build-up

● prevents the progression of renal dysfunction stages

● Decreases the likelihood of developing other chronic health problems, e.g., heart disorders

● has a mild antioxidant function in the body, which keeps inflammation and inflammatory responses under control.

14

The benefits mentioned above are noticeable once the patient follows the diet for at least a month and then continuing it for longer periods to avoid the stage where dialysis is needed. The diet's strictness depends on the current stage of renal/kidney disease if, for example, if you are in the 3rd or 4th stage, you should follow a stricter diet and be attentive to the food, which is allowed or prohibited.

Nutrients You Need

Potassium

Potassium is a naturally occurring mineral found in nearly all foods in varying amounts. Our bodies need an amount of potassium to help with muscle activity as well as electrolyte balance and regulation of blood pressure. However, if potassium is in excess within the system and the kidneys can't expel it (due to renal disease), fluid retention and muscle spasms can occur.

Phosphorus

Phosphorus is a trace mineral found in a wide range of foods and especially dairy, meat, and eggs. It acts synergistically with calcium as well as Vitamin D to promote bone health. However, when there is damage in the kidneys, excess amounts of the mineral cannot be taken out, causing bone weakness.

Calories

When being on a renal diet, it is vital to give yourself the right number of calories to fuel your system. The exact number of calories you should consume daily depends on your age, gender, general health status, and stage of renal disease. In most cases, though, there are no strict limitations in the calorie intake, as long as you take them from proper sources that are low in sodium, potassium, and phosphorus. In general, doctors recommend a daily limit between 1800-2100 calories per day to keep weight within the normal range.

Protein

Protein is an essential nutrient that our systems need to develop and generate new connective tissue, e.g., muscles, even during injuries. Protein also helps stop bleeding and supports the immune system to fight infections. A healthy adult with no kidney disease would usually need 40-65 grams of protein per day.

However, in a renal diet, protein consumption is a tricky subject as too much or too little can cause problems. When metabolized by our systems, protein also creates waste, which is typically processed by the kidneys. However, when kidneys are damaged or underperforming, as in the case of kidney disease, that waste will stay in the system. This is why patients in more advanced CKD stages are advised to limit their protein consumption as well.

Fats

Our systems need fats and particularly good fats as a fuel source and for other metabolic cell functions. A diet high in bad or trans fats can significantly increase the chances of developing heart problems, which often occur with kidney disease. This is why most physicians advise their renal patients to follow a diet that contains a decent amount of good fats and a meager amount of Trans (processed) or saturated fat.

Sodium

Sodium is what our bodies need to regulate fluid and electrolyte balance. It also plays a role in normal cell division in the muscles and nervous system. However, in kidney disease, sodium can quickly spike at higher than normal levels, and the kidneys will be unable to expel it, causing fluid accumulation as a side-effect. Those who also suffer from heart problems as well should limit its consumption as it may raise blood pressure.

Carbohydrates

Carbs act as a major and quick fuel source for the body's cells. When we consume carbs, our systems turn them into glucose and then into energy for "feeding" our body cells. Carbs are generally not restricted in the renal diet. Still, some types of carbs contain dietary fiber as well, which helps regulate normal colon function and protect blood vessels from damage.

Dietary Fiber

Fiber is an important element in our system that cannot be properly digested, but plays a key role in the regulation of our bowel movements and blood cell protection. The fiber in the renal diet is generally encouraged as it helps loosen up the stools, relieve constipation and bloating and protect from colon damage. However, many patients don't get enough amounts of dietary fiber per day, as many of them are high in potassium or phosphorus. Fortunately, there are some good dietary fiber sources for CKD patients that have lower amounts of these minerals compared to others.

Vitamins/Minerals

According to medical research, our systems need at least 13 vitamins and minerals to keep our cells fully active and healthy. However, patients with renal disease are more likely to be depleted by water-soluble vitamins like B-complex and Vitamin C as a result of limited fluid consumption. Therefore, supplementation with these vitamins, along with a renal diet program, should help cover any possible vitamin deficiencies. Supplementation of fat-soluble vitamins like vitamins A, K, and E may be avoided as they can quickly build up in the system and turn toxic.

Fluids

When you are in an advanced stage of renal disease, fluid can quickly build-up and lead to problems. While it is important to keep your system well hydrated, you should avoid minerals like potassium and sodium, which can trigger further fluid build-up and cause a host of other symptoms.

Nutrient You Need to Avoid

Salt or sodium is known for being one of the most important ingredients that the renal diet prohibits its use. This ingredient, although simple, can badly and strongly affect your body, especially the kidneys. Any excess of sodium can't be easily filtered because of the failing condition of the kidneys. A large build-up of sodium can cause catastrophic results on your body. Potassium and Phosphorus are also prohibited for kidney patients depending on the stage of kidney disease.

CHAPTER 2: **BREAKFAST**

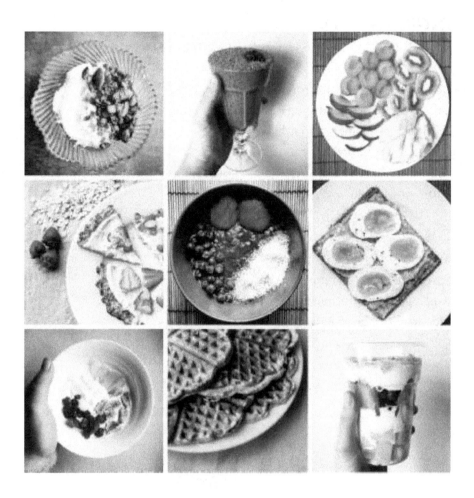

Mediterranean Easy Toast

Prep: 5 mins
Cook: 5 Mins
Servings: 1

INGREDIENTS

4 thick slices whole grain or whole wheat bread of choice
½ cup/123 g hummus
1 cucumber, sliced into rounds
2 tbsp/about 16 g chopped olives of your choice
Za'atar spice blend, to your liking
Handful baby arugula
Crumbled feta cheese, a sprinkle to your liking
1 to 2 Roma tomatoes, sliced into rounds

DIRECTIONS

Toast bread slices to your liking
Spread about 2 tbsp hummus on each slice of bread.
Add a generous sprinkle of Za'atar spice,
then load on the arugula and remaining toppings.

Coconut Flour Pancakes

Prep:15 mins
Cook:15 mins
Servings:6

Ingredients

1 ½ cups coconut flour
½ teaspoon salt
½ cup rice flour
2 teaspoons baking powder
1 teaspoon baking soda
3 cups buttermilk
5 eggs, separated
¼ cup butter, melted
2 teaspoons macadamia nut oil, or more as needed
1 teaspoon almond extract

Directions

Whisk coconut flour, rice flour, baking powder, baking soda, and salt together in a bowl. Mix buttermilk, egg yolks, butter, and almond extract together in a separate bowl.

Heat griddle to 350 degrees F or a skillet over medium-high heat; lightly grease with macadamia nut oil.

Beat egg whites in a glass or metal bowl until medium peaks form. Lift your beater or whisk straight up: the tip of the peak formed by the egg whites should curl over slightly.

Stir buttermilk mixture into flour mixture; fold in egg whites, 1/3 at a time, until batter is just mixed and thick.

Ladle batter onto the griddle and cook until bubbles form and the edges are dry, 3 to 4 minutes. Flip and cook until browned on the other side, 2 to 3 minutes. Repeat with remaining batter.

Nutrition

240 calories
protein 10.2g;
carbohydrates 17.2g
fat 14.6g
cholesterol 180.2mg
sodium 807.5mg.

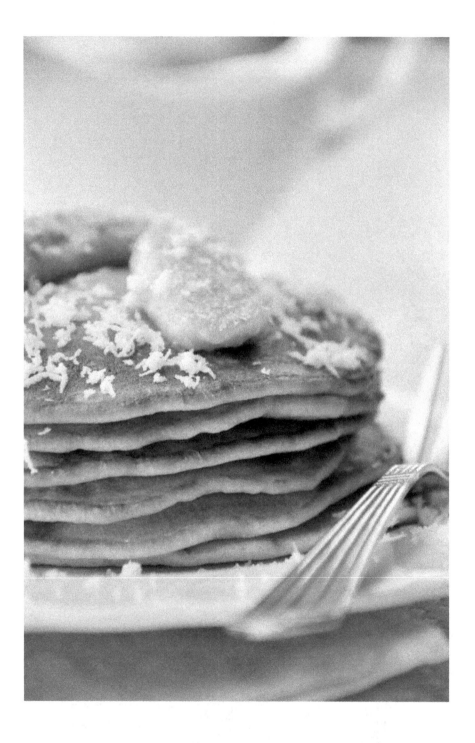

Savoury Buckwheat Granola

Prep:10 mins
Cook:40 mins
Additional:1 hr
Servings:10

Ingredients

2 cups rolled oats
¾ cup buckwheat groats, chopped
1 pinch salt
3 tablespoons coconut oil
¼ cup honey
1 vanilla bean, split and scraped
¾ cup sunflower seeds
½ cup sweetened flaked coconut
½ cup raisins
½ cup almonds, chopped

Directions

oven to 300 degrees F . Line a baking sheet with parchment paper.
  2
Mix oats, buckwheat, sunflower seeds, and salt in a large bowl.
  3
Melt coconut oil in a small saucepan over medium heat; stir in honey
and seeds from vanilla bean until mixed. Pour over oat mixture and
toss to coat. Spread oat mixture evenly over prepared baking sheet.
  4
Bake in the preheated oven, stirring every 10 minutes, until granola is
lightly brown, 35 to 40 minutes. Stir almonds into granola and
continue baking until golden grown, about 5 to 10 minutes more.

Allow granola to cool completely, then stir in coconut and raisins. Store in an airtight container.

Nutrition

304 calories
protein 7.5g
carbohydrates 40g
fat 14.6g
sodium 13.9mg.

Apple Muesli

Prep:10 mins
Cook:20 mins
Servings:4

Ingredients

¾ cup water
½ teaspoon ground cinnamon
¼ cup white sugar
4 apples - peeled, cored and chopped

Directions

In a saucepan, combine apples, water, sugar, and cinnamon. Cover, and cook over medium heat for 18 minutes, or until apples are soft. Allow to cool, then mash with a fork or potato masher.

Nutrition

121 calories;
protein 0.4g;
carbohydrates 31.8g;
fat 0.2g;
sodium 2.7mg

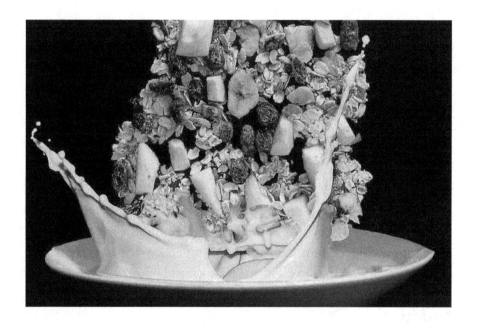

Eggs Creamy Melt

Ingredients

1/2 tablespoon butter

1/8 teaspoon kosher salt, or more to taste

4 large eggs

Directions

Melt the butter in a medium non-stick pan over medium-low heat. Crack eggs into a bowl, add a pinch of salt and whisk until well blended.

When the butter begins to bubble, pour in the eggs and immediately use a silicone spatula to swirl in small circles around the pan, without stopping, until the eggs look slightly thickened and very small curds begin to form, about 30 seconds.

Change from making circles to making long sweeps across the pan until you see larger, creamy curds; about 30 seconds.

When the eggs are softly set and slightly runny in places, remove the pan from the heat and leave for a few seconds to finish cooking. Give a final stir and serve immediately. Serve with an extra sprinkle of salt, a grind of black pepper and a few fresh chopped herbs.

Nutrition

Calories 168 / Protein 13 g / Carbohydrate 1 g / Dietary Fiber 0 g / Total Sugars 0 g / Total Fat 12 g / Saturated Fat 5 g / Cholesterol 380 mg

Master Vanilla Scones

Servings:8

Ingredients

2 cups all-purpose flour

⅓ cup sugar

¼ teaspoon baking soda

½ teaspoon salt

8 tablespoons unsalted butter, frozen

1 teaspoon baking powder

½ cup sour cream

1 large egg

½ cup raisins

Directions

Adjust oven rack to lower-middle position and preheat oven to 400 degrees.

2

In a medium bowl, mix flour, 1/3 cup sugar, baking powder, baking soda and salt. Grate butter into flour mixture on the large holes of a box grater; use your fingers to work in butter (mixture should resemble coarse meal), then stir in raisins.

3

In a small bowl, whisk sour cream and egg until smooth.

4

Using a fork, stir sour cream mixture into flour mixture until large dough clumps form. Use your hands to press the dough against the bowl into a ball. (The dough will be sticky in places, and there may not seem to be enough liquid at first, but as you press, the dough will come together.)

5

Place on a lightly floured surface and pat into a 7- to 8-inch circle about 3/4-inch thick. Sprinkle with remaining 1 tsp. of sugar. Use a sharp knife to cut into 8 triangles; place on a cookie sheet (preferably lined with parchment paper), about 1 inch apart. Bake until golden, about 17 minutes. Cool for 5 minutes and serve warm or at room temperature.

Nutrition

319 calories;
protein 4.9g;
carbohydrates 41.1g;
fat 15.5g;
cholesterol 60.1mg;
sodium 249.3mg.

Creamy Radish Soup

Prep:15 mins
Cook:45 mins
Servings:6

Ingredients

2 tablespoons butter
1 large onion, diced
4 cups raw radish greens
4 cups chicken broth
⅓ cup heavy cream
5 radishes, sliced
2 medium potatoes, sliced

Directions

Melt butter in a large saucepan over medium heat. Stir in the onion, and saute until tender. Mix in the potatoes and radish greens, coating them with the butter. Pour in chicken broth. Bring the mixture to a boil. Reduce heat, and simmer 30 minutes.

2
Allow the soup mixture to cool slightly, and transfer to a blender. Blend until smooth.

3
Return the mixture to the saucepan. Mix in the heavy cream. Cook and stir until well blended. Serve with radish slices.

Nutrition

166 calories; protein 3.8g; carbohydrates 17.9g; fat 9.3g; cholesterol 31.6mg; sodium 688.1mg.

Chia Bars

Prep:15 mins
Cook:30 mins
Additional:8 hrs 10 mins
Servings:24

Ingredients

4 cups water, divided
2 teaspoons salt
2 cups chopped almonds
cooking spray
3 cups all-purpose flour
⅔ cup chocolate chips
⅔ cup olive oil
1 pinch salt
⅔ cup chia seeds
½ cup powdered peanut butter (such as PB2®)
1 tablespoon ground cinnamon
2 teaspoons vanilla extract
½ cup honey

Directions

Combine 2 cup water, almonds, and 1 pinch salt together in a bowl; let sit for 8 hours to overnight. Drain and rinse 2 times.

2

Blend drained almonds and 2 cups water together in a blender until smooth, about 2 minutes. Transfer to a large bowl.

3

Preheat oven to 350 degrees F (175 degrees C). Spray an 11x15-inch baking dish with cooking spray.

4

Mix flour, chocolate chips, olive oil, chia seeds, honey, powdered peanut butter, cinnamon, vanilla extract, and 2 teaspoons salt into almond mixture until dough is evenly combined. Transfer dough to the prepared baking dish, leveling dough with a fork or spatula.
   5
Bake in the preheated oven until cooked through and lightly browned, 35 - 45 minutes. Allow to cool for 10 minutes before cutting into bars.

Nutrition

248 calories;
protein 5.5g;
carbohydrates 25.8g;
fat 14.8g;
sodium 215.1mg.

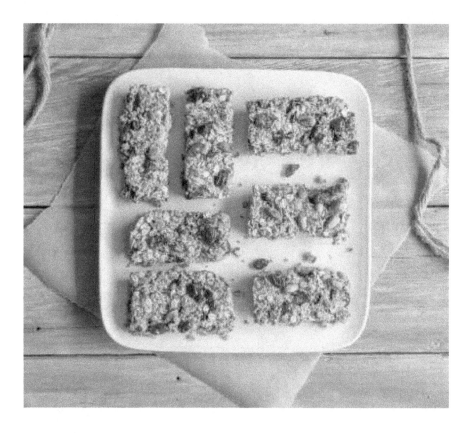

Banana Apple Smoothie

Prep:5 mins
Servings:2

Ingredients

1 frozen bananas, peeled and chopped
1 Gala apple, peeled, cored and chopped
½ cup orange juice
¼ cup milk

Directions

In a blender combine frozen banana, orange juice, apple and milk. Blend until smooth. pour into glasses and serve.

Nutrition

132 calories; protein 2.3g; carbohydrates 30.9g; fat 1g; cholesterol 2.4mg; sodium 14.4mg.

Greek Yogurt

Prep:

10 mins

Additional:

6 mins

Total:

16 mins

Servings:

6

Yield:

6 servings

Ingredients

coffee filters, or as needed
1 (32 ounce) container plain yogurt

Directions

1

Line a colander with coffee filters and set it in a large bowl. Add yogurt and cover with a clean kitchen towel. Place in the refrigerator for 6 hours to overnight; the fluid from the yogurt will collect in the bottom of the bowl.

2

Scoop yogurt out of the coffee filters and back into the original container for storage. Discard accumulated fluid or reserve for other use.

Nutritions

Per Serving: 95 calories; protein 7.9g; carbohydrates 10.7g; fat 2.3g; cholesterol 9.1mg; sodium 105.9mg.

Derby Pie

Prep:

15 mins

Cook:

44 mins

Additional:

30 mins

Total:

1 hr 29 mins

Servings:

8

Yield:

1 9-inch pie

Ingredients

1 (9 inch) store-bought pie crust, unbaked

3 tablespoons bourbon whiskey

¾ teaspoon instant coffee granules

¾ cup chopped pecans

¾ cup white sugar

3 eggs

¾ cup white corn syrup

6 tablespoons butter, melted

1 ½ teaspoons vanilla extract

¾ cup semisweet chocolate chips

Directions

1

Preheat oven to 425 degrees F (220 degrees C).

2

Press pie crust into a 9-inch pie plate. Prick the bottom of the crust with a fork.

3

Bake pie crust in the preheated oven until it looks dry, 4 to 5 minutes. Let cool. Reduce oven temperature to 350 degrees F (175 degrees C).

4

Pour bourbon whiskey into a small pot; heat over very low heat. Stir in instant coffee until dissolved. Stir in pecans.

5

Beat sugar and eggs together in a bowl until well blended. Beat in corn syrup, melted butter, and vanilla extract. Fold in pecan mixture and chocolate chips. Pour mixture into the pie crust.

6

Bake in the preheated oven until filling is firm and golden brown and crust is lightly browned, 40 to 45 minutes. Cool completely before slicing, at least 30 minutes.

Nutritions
Per Serving: 539 calories; protein 5.4g; carbohydrates 64.3g; fat 30.1g; cholesterol 92.6mg; sodium 225.4mg.

CHAPTER 3: LUNCH

BAKED HADDOCK

Prep:10 mins
Cook:15 mins
Servings:4

Ingredients

¾ cup milk
2 teaspoons salt
¼ cup grated Parmesan cheese
4 haddock fillets
¼ cup butter, melted
¼ teaspoon ground dried thyme
¾ cup bread crumbs

Directions

Preheat oven to 500 degrees F .
   2
In a small bowl, combine the milk and salt. In a separate bowl, mix together the bread crumbs, Parmesan cheese, and thyme. Dip the haddock fillets in the milk, then press into the crumb mixture to coat. Place haddock fillets in a glass baking dish, and drizzle with melted butter.
   3
Bake on the top rack of the preheated oven until the fish flakes easily, about 15 minutes.

Nutrition

325 calories; protein 27.7g; carbohydrates 17g; fat 15.7g; cholesterol 103.3mg; sodium 1565.2mg.

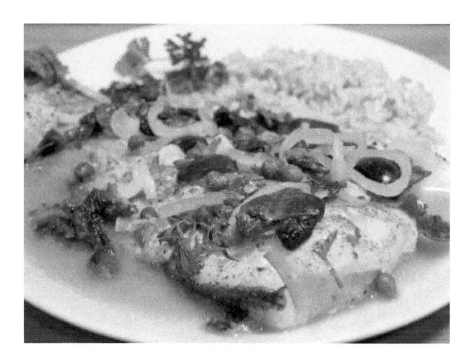

Tzatziki

Prep:20 mins
Additional:6 hrs
Servings:32

Ingredients

32 ounces plain yogurt
¼ cup extra virgin olive oil
5 cloves garlic, minced
3 tablespoons distilled white vinegar
1 large English cucumber, peeled and shredded
salt to taste

Directions

Place a cheese cloth over a medium bowl and strain the yogurt 6 hours in the refrigerator, or over night.
    2
Drain as much excess liquid from the cucumber and garlic as possible.
    3
In a large bowl, mix together the yogurt, cucumber, garlic, vinegar, olive oil and salt. Stir until a thick mixture has formed.

Nutrition

35 calories; protein 1.6g; carbohydrates 2.4g; fat 2.2g; cholesterol 1.7mg; sodium 19.9mg.

Avocado and Mango Salad

Prep:30 mins
Servings:8

Ingredients

Dressing:
½ cup white wine vinegar
¼ cup sunflower seed oil
ground black pepper
4 ripe avocados, cubed
1 teaspoon white sugar
2 mango, cubed
lemons, juiced
2 teaspoons dry mustard
1 head iceberg lettuce, torn, or to taste
1 ½ cups walnut halves
6 slices crispy cooked bacon, crumbled

Directions

Combine vinegar, oil, sugar, mustard, and pepper in a bowl. Refrigerate dressing until ready to serve.
   2
Place avocados, mangoes, and lemon juice in a bowl. Mix gently until just combined.
   3
Place lettuce in a large bowl or platter. Add avocado-mango mixture, walnuts, bacon, and the dressing. Toss and serve.

Nutrition

486 calories; protein 10.1g; carbohydrates 28.6g; fat 40.6g; cholesterol 9.9mg; sodium 225.4mg.

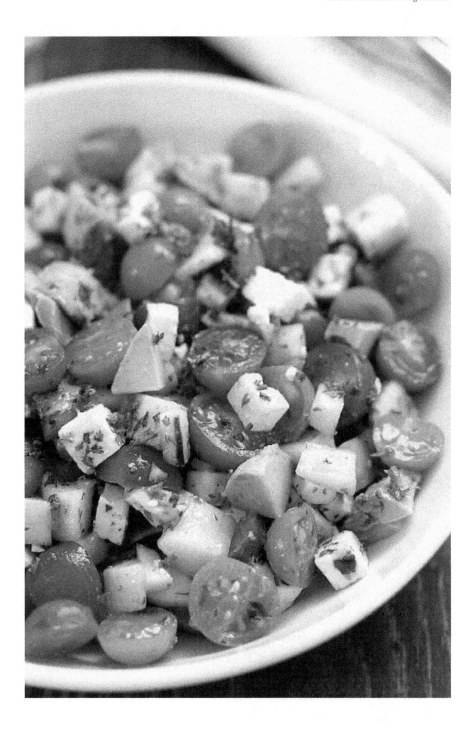

Turmeric and Broccoli Soup

Prep:25 mins
Cook:30 mins
Additional:10 mins
Servings:6

Ingredients

1 ½ pounds broccoli florets and stems
3 tablespoons extra-virgin olive oil
1 carrot, diced
1 large clove garlic, minced
1 onion, diced
1 ½ tablespoons minced fresh ginger
1 teaspoon turmeric powder
½ cup diced red bell pepper
½ teaspoon cracked black pepper
¾ cup plain yogurt
1 (32 ounce) carton low-sodium chicken broth

Directions

Remove broccoli florets from stems and set aside. Trim leaves and set aside. Cut away and discard the tough outer portion of the stems. Dice the remaining cores.

   2

Turn on a multi-functional pressure cooker,

Nutrition

151 calories; protein 7.4g; carbohydrates 14.5g; fat 8g; cholesterol 4.4mg; sodium 138.7mg.

Winter Citrus Salad

Prep:30 mins
Servings:6

Ingredients

Dressing:
½ cup canola oil
¼ cup apple cider vinegar
½ cup white sugar
2 tablespoons sesame oil
2 tablespoons toasted sesame seeds
1 teaspoon minced garlic
2 tablespoons poppy seeds
½ teaspoon ground paprika
2 tablespoons minced onion
Salad:
1 (12 ounce) bag mixed salad greens
¼ cup chopped green onions
1 (8 ounce) can mandarin oranges, drained
½ cup toasted sliced almonds
¼ cup crumbled Gorgonzola cheese
½ cup grape tomatoes

Directions

Combine canola oil, sugar, apple cider vinegar, sesame oil, onion, poppy seeds, sesame seeds, garlic, and paprika in a jar. Close and shake jar until dressing is well mixed.
Place salad greens in a large bowl. Pour in half of the dressing; toss to mix. Arrange mandarin oranges, grape tomatoes, almonds, Gorgonzola cheese, and green onions on top.

Nutrition

404 calories; protein 5.2g; carbohydrates 26.3g; fat 31.7g; cholesterol 6mg; sodium 75.7mg.

ITALIAN prosciutto wraps mozzarella balls

INGREDIENTS

Marinara Sauce 750g
Baguette 750 1 sliced
¼ Butter, softened
2 minced/ grated Cloves garlic
1 Pound Mozzarella Balls
1 Tablespoon Olive Oil
¼ cup grated (optional)
6 ounces, cut in half Prosciutto

Directions:

Spread the mixture of the butter and garlic over the baguette slices and toast until lightly golden brown.

Meanwhile, wrap the mozzarella in prosciutto.

Heat the oil in a pan over medium-high heat, add the prosciutto wrapped mozzarella and cook until lightly golden brown, about a minute per side, and set aside.

Add Pomì Marinara Sauce and parmesan to the pan and heat until the cheese has melted in.

Add the prosciutto wrapped mozzarella and transfer to a preheated 425F oven to bake until the sauce is bubbling and the mozzarella has melted, about 5-10 minutes, before removing from the oven, sprinkling on the basil and enjoying with the garlic crostini.

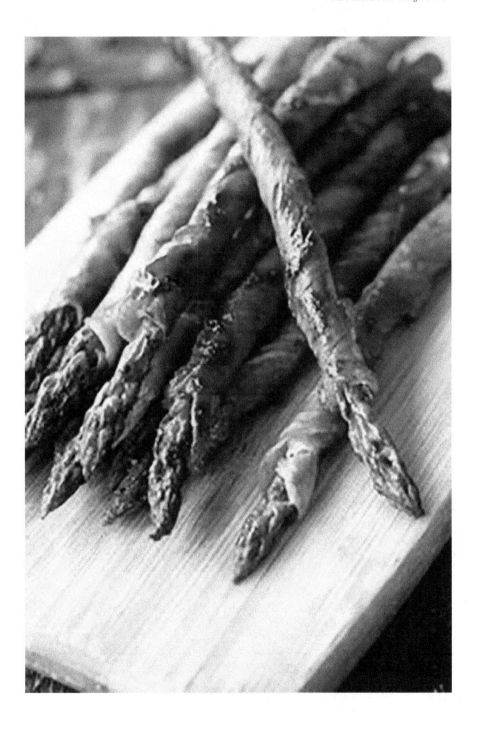

Macaroni & Cheese

Prep:10 mins
Cook:12 mins
Servings:4

Ingredients

1 (6 ounce) box Macaroni & Mild Cheddar Cheese
½ cup shredded sharp Cheddar cheese
2 ounces Organic Milk
1 cup Cooked broccoli florets
1 tablespoon butter

Directions

Cook the noodles according to the package directions.
Drain and pour into a large bowl.
Immediately add the butter and shredded cheese. Stir to mix while still
hot. The cheese should melt. If it doesn't, put the mixture back in the
pan and heat for another minute on medium, stirring constantly until
the cheese has melted.
Add the cheese mix, milk, and broccoli, if using. Stir until combined.

Nutrition

255 calories; protein 10.1g; carbohydrates 33g; fat 9.3g; cholesterol
24.6mg; sodium 482.2mg.

Honey Molasses Pork

Serves:6
Prep:2 Hr 10 Min
Cook: 30 Min

Directions

In a bowl combine all ingredients except pork chops, stir well. In a large bowl put the chops and pour marinade over the top, making sure to cover them all. Every 1/2 move them around in the marinade. Marinade 2hr or longer.

Turn grill to medium. Place chops on a grill pan and cook 16-20 minutes or until done. Through out grilling, brush marinade over chops.

Giblet Gravy

Prep:10 mins
Cook:2 hrs 15 mins
Servings:16

Ingredients

1 turkey neck and giblets
2 large white onions, sliced
1 cup sliced carrots
1 cup dry white wine
½ cup celery leaves
6 cloves garlic, peeled
6 cups chicken broth
½ cup turkey drippings
¾ cup all-purpose flour
6 tablespoons butter, softened
1 bay leaf
salt and ground black pepper to taste

Directions

Cut turkey neck in half. Set liver aside.
Combine neck, giblets, broth, onions, carrots, wine, celery, garlic, and bay leaf in a pot. Bring to a boil. Reduce heat and simmer for 1 hour and 30 minutes. Add liver and simmer for 30 minutes more.
Mix flour and butter together to form a thick paste.
Remove and discard neck and giblets. Strain broth, pressing vegetables to extract liquid. Discard vegetables. Add turkey drippings. Add flour mixture gradually and stir until smooth. Bring to a boil and cook until desired thickness is reached, 8 to 10 minutes. Season with salt and pepper.

Nutrition

180 calories; protein 4.7g; carbohydrates 8.4g; fat 12.9g; cholesterol 64.3mg; sodium 496.7mg.

Bread Fondue

Servings:

20

Yield:

1 - 9 inch ring

Ingredients

3 ½ teaspoons white sugar

2 teaspoons salt

1 tablespoon active dry yeast

4 cups all-purpose flour

½ cup margarine

1 cup milk

1 egg

1 egg yolk

2 pounds Muenster cheese, shredded

1 egg white, beaten

2 tablespoons whole blanched almonds

Directions

1

Heat milk and butter or margarine over low heat until very warm.

2

Combine sugar, salt, yeast, and 1 cup of flour in a large bowl. Stir in hot milk mixture, and beat with mixer on medium speed for 2 minutes. Beat in 1 more cup of flour, and continue beating for 2 more minutes. With a wooden spoon, stir in enough flour (about 2 cups) to make a soft dough.

3

Knead the dough on a lightly floured surface for about 10 minutes, adding more flour as necessary. Cover dough with bowl, and let rest for 15 minutes.

4

Meanwhile, shred muenster cheese. Combine with 1 egg and 1 egg yolk.

5

On a lightly floured surface and with a floured rolling pin, roll dough into a 24 x 6 inch rectangle. Spoon the cheese mixture into a log shape lengthwise along the dough. Fold the dough over the cheese making a 1 inch overlap, and pinch seam to seal. In a greased 9 inch round cake pan, place roll, seam side down, to make a ring. Overlap the ends, and pinch to seal. Cover with a towel. Let rest 10 minutes.

6

Brush loaf with egg white, and garnish with blanched almonds, if desired. Bake at 350 degrees F (175 degrees C) for 1 hour, until loaf sounds hollow when tapped. Remove bread from pan immediately. Cool for 15 minutes before slicing into wedges.

Nutritions

Per Serving: 321 calories; protein 14.7g; carbohydrates 21.4g; fat 19.6g; cholesterol 64.1mg; sodium 582.7mg.

Veggie Chili

Prep:
45 mins
Cook:
1 hr
Total:
1 hr 45 mins
Servings:
8
Yield:
8 servings

Ingredients

½ cup texturized vegetable protein (TVP)
1 cup water
2 ½ tablespoons olive oil
1 onion, chopped
6 cloves garlic, minced
1 teaspoon salt
1 teaspoon ground black pepper
2 teaspoons chili powder
2 teaspoons ground cumin
2 teaspoons ground cayenne pepper
¼ teaspoon cinnamon
1 tablespoon honey
2 (12 ounce) cans kidney beans with liquid
2 (12 ounce) cans diced tomatoes with juice
1 green bell pepper, chopped
2 carrots, finely chopped
1 bunch green onions, chopped

1 bunch cilantro, chopped

1 (8 ounce) container dairy sour cream

Directions

1

Place the textured vegetable protein (TVP) in water, and soak 30 minutes. Press to drain.

2

Heat the oil in a large pot over medium heat, and saute TVP, onion, and garlic until onion is tender and TVP is evenly browned. Season with salt, pepper, 1/2 the chili powder, 1/2 the cumin, 1/2 the cayenne pepper, and cinnamon. Mix in honey, beans, tomatoes, green bell pepper, and carrots. Cook, stirring, occasionally, 45 minutes.

3

Season the chili with remaining chili powder, cumin, and cayenne pepper, and continue cooking 15 minutes. To serve, divide into bowls, garnish with green onions and cilantro, and top with dollops of sour cream.

Nutritions

Per Serving: 253 calories; protein 13.3g; carbohydrates 27.2g; fat 11.2g; cholesterol 12.5mg; sodium 718.4mg.

CHAPTER 4: DINNER

Lamb with Spinach

Prep:30 mins
Cook:30 mins
Servings:4

Ingredients

20 potatoes, halved
2 cloves garlic, minced
2 tablespoons brown sugar
1 cup red wine
4 (6 ounce) lamb shoulder steaks
salt and pepper to taste
1 tablespoon butter
1 tablespoon cumin seeds
2 bunches fresh spinach, cleaned
¼ cup sour cream
2 tablespoons softened butter
1 tablespoon vegetable oil

Directions

Place potatoes into a large saucepan and cover with salted water. Bring to a boil, then reduce heat to medium-low, cover, and simmer until tender, about 15 minutes. Drain and allow to steam dry for a minute or two.

Melt the butter in a saucepan over medium heat. Stir in the garlic, and cook for 3 to 4 minutes until the aroma of the garlic has mellowed. Add the brown sugar and red wine, then bring to a boil over medium-high heat. Allow to boil for 5 minutes, then remove from the heat, cover, and keep warm.

Meanwhile, season the lamb steaks with salt and pepper to taste. Press the cumin seeds into the steaks on both sides. Heat the vegetable oil in a large skillet over medium-high heat. Add the steaks, and cook on both sides until cooked to your desired degree of doneness, about 4 minutes per side for medium. Remove the steaks to rest in a warm spot. Place the spinach into the hot skillet, season to taste with salt and pepper, and cook until the spinach has wilted.

Mash the potatoes with the sour cream and butter; season to taste with salt and pepper. To serve, mound a serving of mashed potatoes onto the center of a dinner plate. Top with the spinach and a lamb steak. Strain the red wine sauce overtop.

Nutrition

1063 calories; protein 43.3g; carbohydrates 96.5g; fat 53g; cholesterol 151.6mg; sodium 341.7mg.

Turmeric Tilapia

Servings: 24

Ingredients

1 thumb
Ginger
1 Unit Lime
¼ ounce Cilantro
1 unit Shallot
2 clove Garlic
½ cup Jasmine Rice
1 tablespoon Brown Sugar
6 ounce Green Beans
11 ounce Tilapia
1 teaspoon Turmeric
¼ cup Shredded Coconut
1 unit Veggie Stock Concentrate

Directions

Wash and dry all produce (except green beans). Peel and grate or mince ginger. Zest and quarter lime (zest 1 lime; quarter both for 4 servings). Chop cilantro leaves and stems. Halve and peel shallot; mince one half (mince both halves for 4). Mince half the garlic (mince all the garlic for 4).

In a small pot, combine rice, ¾ cup water (1½ cups for 4 servings), brown sugar, and ½ tsp salt (1 tsp for 4). Bring to a boil, then cover and reduce to a low simmer. Cook until rice is tender, 16-18 minutes. Keep covered off heat until ready to serve.

Meanwhile, heat a large, preferably nonstick, pan over medium-high heat. Add coconut and cook, stirring constantly, until golden brown, 2-3 minutes. Transfer to a plate. Turn off heat and wipe out pan.

Pierce green bean bag with a fork; place bag on a plate. Microwave until tender, 1-2 minutes. (TIP: No microwave? No problem! Steam beans in a small pot with a splash of water until just tender, 6-8 minutes.) Transfer to a medium bowl and toss with 1 TBSP butter until melted. Season with salt and pepper. Keep covered until ready to serve.

Pat tilapia dry with paper towels; season generously with salt and pepper. Rub all over with turmeric. Heat a large drizzle of oil in pan used for coconut over medium-high heat. Add tilapia; cook until firm and cooked through, 4-6 minutes per side. Turn off heat; transfer to a plate. Wipe out pan. Heat a drizzle of oil in same pan over medium heat. Add ginger, shallot, and garlic; cook, stirring, until fragrant, 1 minute. Stir in ¼ cup water (⅓ cup for 4), stock concentrate, and juice from half the lime. Simmer until slightly reduced, 2-3 minutes. Turn off heat.

Add 2 TBSP butter to pan with sauce. Stir in half the cilantro and season with salt and pepper. Fluff rice; stir in 1 TBSP butter, coconut, and lime zest. Divide rice, green beans, and tilapia between plates. Spoon sauce over tilapia. Sprinkle with remaining cilantro. Serve with remaining lime wedges on the side.

Nutrition
Energy (kJ)3012 kJ
Calories720 kcal
Fat39 g
Saturated Fat11 g
Carbohydrate61 g
Sugar10 g
Dietary Fiber5 g
Protein34 g
Cholesterol125 mg
Sodium560 mg

Crispy Fish Fillets

Prep:10 mins
Cook:10 mins
Servings:4

Ingredients

1 egg
4 (6 ounce) fillets sole
½ teaspoon salt
1 ½ cups instant mashed potato flakes
¼ cup oil for frying
2 tablespoons prepared yellow mustard

Directions

In a shallow dish, whisk together the egg, mustard, and salt; set aside.
Place the potato flakes in another shallow dish.
Heat oil in a large heavy skillet over medium-high heat.
Dip fish fillets in the egg mixture. Dredge the fillets in the potato
flakes, making sure to completely coat the fish. For extra crispy, dip
into egg and potato flakes again.
Fry fish fillets in oil for 3 to 4 minutes on each side, or until golden
brown.

Nutrition

391 calories; protein 30g; carbohydrates 26.2g; fat 18.1g; cholesterol
136.8mg; sodium 655.9mg.

Shrimp and Catfish Gumbo

Prep:30 mins
Cook:1 hr
Servings:10

Ingredients

¼ cup cooking oil
1 bell pepper, chopped
2 cloves garlic, minced
1 large onion, chopped
4 cubes beef bouillon
2 stalks celery, chopped
1 (16 ounce) package frozen sliced okra
4 cups shrimp, peeled and deveined
6 cups hot water
1 (28 ounce) can diced tomatoes, undrained
¼ teaspoon cayenne pepper
½ teaspoon dried thyme
2 teaspoons salt
2 bay leaves
2 pounds catfish fillets, cut into 1 inch pieces
1 teaspoon dry crab boil

Directions

Warm oil in a skillet over medium heat. Stir in onion, bell pepper, celery, and garlic. Cook until soft, about 10 minutes.
Dissolve bouillon cubes in hot water. Pour into skillet. Stir tomatoes, okra, and shrimp into skillet. Season with salt, cayenne pepper, thyme, bay leaves, and crab boil. Bring to a boil; cover, and simmer 30 minutes.

Place fish in skillet, return to boil; cover, and simmer 15 minutes more. Remove bay leaves, and serve.

Nutrition

269 calories; protein 26.5g; carbohydrates 8.8g; fat 13.5g; cholesterol 120.6mg; sodium 1030mg.

Sorrel Soup

Prep:10 mins
Cook:10 mins
Servings:6

Ingredients

2 tablespoons uncooked white rice
salt and pepper to taste
1 bunch sorrel, stemmed and rinsed
½ cup heavy cream
3 cups vegetable broth

Directions

In a large saucepan, bring broth to a boil over medium-high heat. Stir in rice, reduce heat, and simmer for about 8 minutes. Stir in sorrel and return to a boil. Remove from heat and puree in batches in a blender or food processor or using an immersion blender.
Return to medium-low heat and stir in cream, salt, and pepper. Heat through and serve.

Nutrition

112 calories; protein 1.5g; carbohydrates 9.5g; fat 7.8g; cholesterol 27.2mg; sodium 239.3mg.

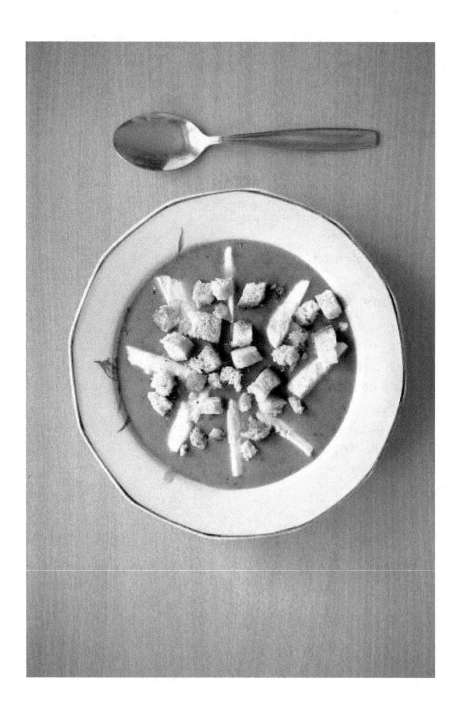

Linguine Shrimps & Garlic

Prep:10 mins
Cook:20 mins
Servings:4

Ingredients

1 (16 ounce) package fresh linguine pasta
1 pound large shrimp, peeled and deveined
3 tablespoons chopped fresh basil
3 tablespoons olive oil, divided
 tablespoons butter, cut up
¼ cup grated Asiago cheese
2 teaspoons minced garlic

Directions

Bring a large pot of lightly salted water and 1 tablespoon oil to a boil.
Cook linguine in the boiling water, stirring occasionally, until tender
yet firm to the bite, about 8 minutes. Drain and set aside.
Heat remaining olive oil in a large skillet over medium-high heat. Add
shrimp and saute until shrimp turns pink, 3 to 4 minutes. Add basil
and garlic; cook for 2 to 3 minutes more.
Add butter and cooked linguine. Toss until butter melts, making sure
to coat the linguine with the sauce. Remove from heat. Serve
immediately.

Nutrition

729 calories; protein 33.5g; carbohydrates 72g; fat 34.2g; cholesterol
267.3mg; sodium 477.4mg.

Jamaican Curried Goat

Prep:15 mins
Cook:1 hr 44 mins
Additional:1 hr
Servings:8

Ingredients

2 pounds goat stew meat, cut into 1-inch cubes
2 tablespoons curry powder
2 cloves garlic, minced
2 fresh hot chile peppers, seeded and chopped
1 teaspoon salt
3 tablespoons vegetable oil
1 onion, chopped
1 teaspoon ground black pepper
1 rib celery, chopped
2 ½ cups vegetable broth
3 potatoes, peeled and cut into 1-inch chunks
1 bay leaf

Directions

Combine goat meat, chile pepper, curry powder, garlic, salt, and black pepper in a bowl. Cover and refrigerate to allow flavors to blend, 1 hour to overnight.

Remove goat meat mixture from bowl and pat dry, reserving marinade. Heat vegetable oil in a stockpot over medium-high heat. Cook meat in batches, browning on all sides, 4 to 6 minutes per batch. Transfer meat to a plate. Add onion and celery to the stockpot; cook and stir until onion begins to brown, 4 to 6 minutes.

Stir browned goat meat into onion mixture. Add reserved marinade, vegetable broth, and bay leaf. Bring to a boil, cover, reduce heat to low, and simmer for 1 hour. Stir in potatoes; simmer until potatoes and meat are tender, 35 to 45 minutes more.

Remove stockpot from heat, skim off surface fat, and remove bay leaf.

Nutrition

238 calories; protein 21.9g; carbohydrates 20.1g; fat 7.8g; cholesterol 53.2mg; sodium 509.3mg.

Shredded Chicken

Prep:5 mins
Cook:3 hrs
Servings:12

Ingredients

1 cup chicken broth
½ teaspoon seasoned salt, or to taste
3 pounds skinless, boneless chicken breast halves

Directions

Place chicken breasts in the bottom of a slow cooker. Pour in chicken broth and seasoned salt. Cover and cook on High until no longer pink in the center and the juices run clear, 3 to 4 hours, or on Low for 6 to 8 hours. An instant-read thermometer inserted into the center of the chicken breasts should read at least 165 degrees F .
Remove chicken and shred with 2 forks.

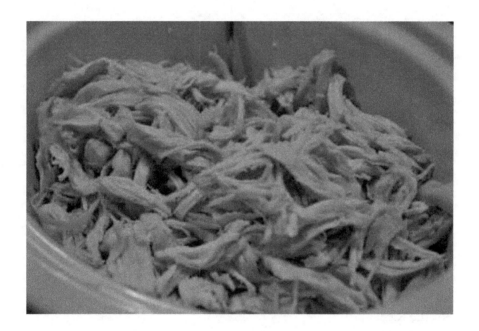

Exotic Palabok

Prep:30 mins
Cook:1 hr
Additional:4 hrs 10 mins
Servings:8

Ingredients

For the Exotic Marinade:
⅓ cup plain yogurt
1 medium lime, zested and juiced
2 teaspoons kosher salt
1 teaspoon ground paprika
1 teaspoon ground cumin
½ teaspoon ground coriander
¼ teaspoon cayenne pepper
¼ teaspoon ground white pepper
¼ teaspoon ground cinnamon
¼ teaspoon ground allspice
1 (2 to 3 pound) whole chicken, cut into 8 pieces
¼ teaspoon ground cardamom

For the Rice:
1 pinch saffron
2 ¼ cups chicken broth, divided
2 tablespoons unsalted butter
1 ½ cups basmati rice
1 drizzle olive oil
1 teaspoon kosher salt
salt to taste

Directions

Add yogurt, lime zest and juice, salt, paprika, cumin, coriander, cayenne, white pepper, cardamom, cinnamon, and allspice for marinade to a large mixing bowl; whisk to combine.

Make one or two slits into each piece of dark chicken meat, down to the bone. Add chicken parts to the yogurt marinade and toss very thoroughly. Wrap in plastic wrap and marinate in the refrigerator for 4 to 8 hours.

Preheat the oven to 450 degrees F. Lightly grease a 9x13-inch casserole dish.

Grind saffron in a mortar with a pestle. Pour in 1/4 cup chicken broth and stir to combine.

Combine unsalted butter and salt in a saucepan; pour in remaining 2 cups chicken broth and chicken broth-saffron mixture. Bring to a boil over high heat. Add basmati rice and stir to combine. Reduce heat to low, cover tightly, and let simmer gently for exactly 15 minutes; do not disturb while cooking. Turn off the heat and let rest for 10 minutes. While rice is still hot, transfer into the prepared casserole dish. Use a fork to fluff the rice while gently spreading into an even layer. Place the chicken pieces, skin-side up, on top of rice. Drizzle with olive oil and sprinkle with salt.

Roast in the center of the preheated oven until chicken is no longer pink in the centers and juices run clear, about 45 minutes. An instant-read thermometer inserted into the thickest part of the thigh, near the bone, should read 165 degrees F .

While chicken is in the oven, mix yogurt, garlic, green onions, mint, cilantro, salt, and water together for sauce. Reserve in the refrigerator until needed. Serve chicken and rice on a plate and top with sauce.

Nutrition

362 calories; protein 23.8g; carbohydrates 31.7g; fat 15.4g; cholesterol 71.5mg; sodium 1125.5mg.

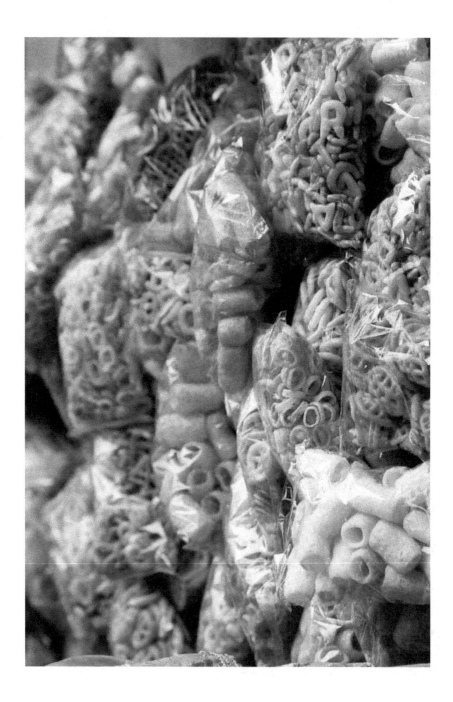

Romesco Sauce

Prep:

10 mins

Cook:

25 mins

Additional:

10 mins

Total:

45 mins

Servings:

10

Yield:

2 1/2 cups

Ingredients

6 roma (plum) tomatoes, halved

1 large red bell pepper, quartered

12 cloves garlic

⅔ cup olive oil

kosher salt to taste

1 slice bread

½ cup toasted whole almonds

½ cup red wine vinegar

½ teaspoon Spanish paprika

1 pinch crushed red pepper flakes, or to taste

Directions

1

Preheat an oven to 425 degrees F (220 degrees C). Line a baking sheet with aluminum foil.

2

Place the tomatoes, bell pepper, and garlic cloves onto the prepared baking sheet. Brush the vegetables with some of the olive oil, then sprinkle with kosher salt. Bake in the preheated oven until the garlic has turned golden brown, 15 to 20 minutes. Remove from the oven, and allow to cool for 10 minutes. While the vegetables are cooling, bake the bread slice on one of the oven racks until golden brown. Remove and allow to cool.

3

Scrape the vegetables and any juices from the pan into a food processor or blender. Break the bread into pieces, and add to the food processor along with the toasted almonds, vinegar, paprika, and red pepper flakes. Puree until finely ground, then drizzle in the remaining olive oil with the machine running. Season to taste with additional salt if necessary.

Nutritions
Per Serving: 196 calories; protein 2.4g; carbohydrates 7.3g; fat 18.3g; sodium 60.6mg.

Cucumber Soup

Prep:

15 mins

Additional:

30 mins

Total:

45 mins

Servings:

4

Yield:

4 servings

Ingredients

4 cucumbers - peeled, quartered, and seeded

1 (14.5 ounce) can chicken broth

1 cup chopped tomato

¼ cup fresh lime juice

⅛ teaspoon cayenne pepper

Directions

1

Place 2 cucumbers in a blender; pour in chicken stock. Blend cucumber mixture until smooth and pureed; pour cucumber puree into a large bowl.

2

Chop the remaining 2 cucumbers. Stir chopped cucumbers, tomato, lime juice, and cayenne pepper into pureed cucumber until well mixed. Refrigerate until chilled, at least 30 minutes.

Nutritions

Per Serving: 43 calories; protein 2.1g; carbohydrates 8.6g; fat 0.7g; cholesterol 2.3mg; sodium 441.6mg.

CHAPTER 5: SNACKS AND SIDES RECIPES

Pecan Caramel Corn

yield: 30 SERVINGS
prep time: 30 MINUTES
cook time: 2 HOURS
additional time: 30 MINUTES

INGREDIENTS

15-18 cups popcorn
3/4 teaspoon baking soda
2 cups raw whole pecans
1 1/2 cups brown sugar
1/2 cup light corn syrup
1/4 teaspoon salt
3/4 cups salted butter

DIRECTIONS

Preheat oven to 225 degrees.

Prepare 15-18 cups of plain popcorn. Place popcorn in a large roasting pan and sprinkle 2 cups of raw whole pecans on top of the popcorn.

Heat salted butter, brown sugar, light corn syrup, and salt in a medium heavy saucepan over medium heat. Stir continually with a wooden spoon until the ingredients are melted and well-combined.

Once bubbles begin forming around the edges, cook over medium heat for 5 minutes, without stirring.

Remove from heat and add 3/4 teaspoon of baking soda. Stir until foamy.

Pour the foaming caramel sauce over the prepared popcorn and nuts and stir together until the popcorn and nuts are evenly coated with caramel.

Spread evenly in the roasting pan and bake for 2 hours in the heated oven, stirring every 20 minutes.

Turn over onto wax paper and allow to cool completely, for about 30 minutes.

Store in an airtight containter for up to 3 weeks.

Nutrition Information

Yield30Serving Size1Amount Calories535Total Fat34gSaturated Fat8gTrans Fat7gUnsaturated Fat22gCholesterol12mgSodium635mgCarbohydrates53gFiber8gSugar14gProtein6g

Citrus Salad Sauce

Prep Time: 10 minutes
Cook Time: 0 minutes
Yield: About 3/4 cup 1x

INGREDIENTS

2 tablespoons orange juice, plus zest of 1/2 orange
1/2 cup olive oil
1/2 tablespoon Dijon mustard
1 tablespoon lemon juice
1/2 teaspoon maple syrup
Fresh ground black pepper
1/4 teaspoon kosher salt

DIRECTIONS

Zest the orange. In a medium bowl, mix the orange juice, orange zest, lemon juice, mustard, maple syrup, salt and a grind of fresh black pepper.
Gradually whisk in the olive oil 1 tablespoon at a time (8 tablespoons total), until creamy and emulsified. If desired, season with additional salt.

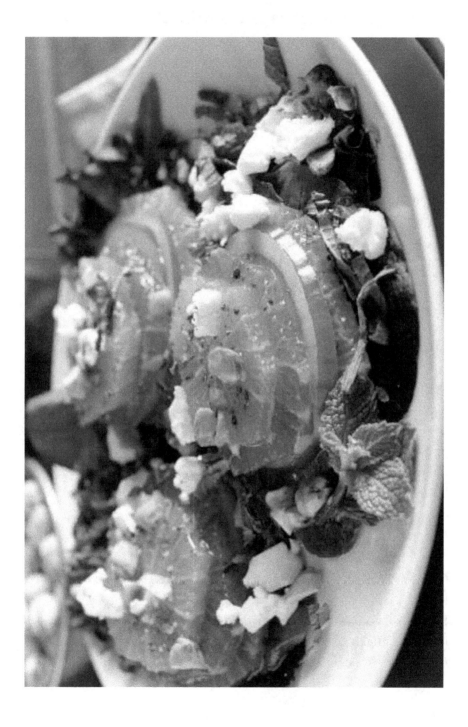

Mini Zucchini Pizza Bites Mini Zucchini Pà

Pizza BitesPrep Time10 mins
 Cook Time10 mins
 Servings6 servings

Ingredients

2 large zucchini
1 teaspoon oregano
½ cup low carb pizza or tomato sauce
2 cups mozzarella cheese
pizza toppings as desired
¼ cup parmesan cheese

Directions

Preheat oven to 450°F. Line a baking pan with foil and set aside.
Slice Zucchini ¼" thick and arrange on prepared baking sheet.
Top zucchini slices with pizza sauce, oregano, cheese and your favorite
pizza toppings.
Bake 5 min or until zucchini is tender. Broil 5 min or until cheese is
bubbly and melted.

Nutrition

Calories: 145kcal | Carbohydrates: 4g | Protein: 10g | Fat: 9g | Satura
ted
Fat: 5g | Cholesterol: 32mg | Sodium: 413mg | Potassium: 266mg | F
iber: 1g | Sugar: 2g | Vitamin A: 505IU | Vitamin
C: 13.1mg | Calcium: 256mg | Iron: 0.8mg

Fajita Flavor Marinade

Prep:20 mins
Cook:10 mins
Additional:2 hrs
Servings:4

Ingredients

1 pound beef round steak, cut into thin strips
1 yellow bell pepper, cut into thin strips
1 red onion, thinly sliced
2 anaheim chile peppers, thinly sliced
1 red bell pepper, cut into thin strips
6 tablespoons olive oil
4 large cloves garlic, crushed
1 (1.27 ounce) packet spicy fajita seasoning

Directions

Combine beef strips, red bell pepper, yellow bell pepper, onion, anaheim chile peppers, fajita seasoning, olive oil, and garlic in a large bowl. Cover and refrigerate for at least 2 hours.
Heat a large skillet over medium heat; cook and stir the beef and vegetable mixture in hot skillet until beef is no longer pink in the center and vegetables are tender, about 10 minutes.

Nutrition

366 calories; protein 22.9g; carbohydrates 16.4g; fat 23.8g; cholesterol 56.3mg; sodium 659.5mg.

Turmeric Milk

Prep:

10 mins

Cook:

5 mins

Total:

15 mins

Servings:

1

Yield:

1 cup

Ingredients

1 (1 1/2 inch) piece fresh turmeric root, peeled and grated

1 (1/2 inch) piece fresh ginger root, peeled and grated

1 tablespoon honey

1 cup unsweetened almond milk

Directions

1

Combine turmeric root, ginger root, and honey together in a bowl, crushing the turmeric and ginger as much as possible.

2

Heat almond milk in a saucepan over medium-low heat. Once small bubbles begin to form around the edges, reduce heat to low. Transfer about 2 tablespoon milk to turmeric mixture to allow mixture to soften and honey to melt into a paste-like mixture.

3

Mix the turmeric paste into milk in the saucepan; raise temperature to medium-low and cook, stirring continuously, until fully combined. Blend with an immersion blender for a smooth texture.

4

Pour turmeric tea into a mug and top with ground turmeric and cinnamon.

Nutritions

Per Serving: 143 calories; protein 1.5g; carbohydrates 29.3g; fat 2.9g; sodium 162.6mg.

Garlic Oyster Crackers

Prep:

10 mins

Cook:

20 mins

Total:

30 mins

Servings:

24

Yield:

24 servings

Ingredients

¾ cup vegetable oil

1 (1 ounce) package dry Ranch-style dressing mix

½ teaspoon dried dill weed

¼ teaspoon lemon pepper

¼ teaspoon garlic powder

1 (12 ounce) package oyster crackers

Directions

1

Preheat oven to 275 degrees F (135 degrees C).

2

In a mixing bowl, whisk together vegetable oil, ranch-style dressing mix, dill weed, lemon pepper and garlic powder. Pour this spice mixture over the crackers in a medium bowl, and stir until the crackers are coated. Arrange the crackers on a large baking sheet.

3

Bake in the preheated 275 degrees F (135 degrees C) oven for 15 to 20 minutes.

Nutritions

Per Serving: 128 calories; protein 1.1g; carbohydrates 9.7g; fat 9.4g; sodium 354.3mg.

CHAPTER 6: DESSERTS

Chocolate Pudding Cake

Servings:24

Ingredients

1 (10 inch) angel food cake
1 (8 ounce) container frozen whipped topping, thawed
1 (5.9 ounce) package instant chocolate pudding mix
1 (1.55 ounce) bar milk chocolate

Directions

Tear angel food cake into bite size pieces into a 9x13 inch cake pan
(preferably glass).
Prepare chocolate pudding as directed on package. Gently spread over
the top of cake pieces, spreading to edges of pan.
Carefully spread whipped topping over chocolate pudding, spreading
to edges of pan and taking care not to mix with pudding.
Using a cheese grater or vegetable peeler, grate chocolate bar over the
whipped topping.
Chill until ready to serve, at least one hour.

Nutrition

102 calories; protein 1.2g; carbohydrates 17.4g; fat 3.1g; cholesterol
0.4mg; sodium 207mg

Coconut Loaf Cake

Ingredients

The Cake Batter
175 g or ¾ cup softened butter
290 g or 1 ½ cups regular sugar
3 eggs (lightly beaten)
225 g or 1 ¾ cups Plain / All purpose flour (sieved)
175 ml or ¾ cup coconut milk
1 ½ Teaspoons baking powder
6 Tablespoons desiccated / shredded coconut
½ Teaspoon salt

DIRECTIONS

Heat oven to 160c, 300F. Grease and line your baking tin. See here for how to line.

Get all your ingredients ready, i.e coconut, sieve the flour, and add the salt and baking powder to the flour etc.

Start with making the cake batter by creaming the butter and sugar until a pale light color.

Slowly add the beaten eggs to the mixer, on a low-speed setting, a bit at a time. If the mixture starts to curdle or split, add a spoonful of your sieved flour, keep on adding the eggs, and a bit of flour if necessary until all the eggs are added

Add the coconut milk with half of the flour, keeping the mixer on a slow speed. Once combined, add the shredded/desiccated coconut, and the rest of the flour.

Transfer the cake mixture to the greased and lined loaf tin. Then place in the oven for 1 hr and 5 minutes, check after 1 hour.

Have a cup of tea whilst your coconut pound cake is baking and giving off those lovely aromas in your kitchen!

When the cake is done, take it out of the oven and leave in the cake tin until cool. Whilst the cake is still HOT, using a skewer, prick holes all over the top of the cake, pushing the skewer through to the bottom of the cake.

Hazelnut Cake

Servings:36

Ingredients

1 (18.25 ounce) package devil's food cake mix

1 (3.9 ounce) package instant chocolate pudding mix

¼ cup water

3 cups heavy whipping cream

1 teaspoon vanilla extract

1 cup finely chopped toasted hazelnuts

12 hazelnuts

1 ½ cups semisweet chocolate chips

Directions

Prepare cake mix according to package directions, using required ingredients, plus pudding mix, vanilla, and an additional 1/4 cup of water. Spread batter evenly among three greased and floured 9 inch cake pans. Bake at temperature specified on cake mix box for 18 to 22 minutes, or until a toothpick inserted in the center comes out clean. Let cakes cool completely, then chill in refrigerator for 30 minutes. In a double boiler over simmering water, melt chocolate chips. Gradually add 1/4 cup of the whipping cream, stirring constantly until smooth. Remove from heat and let cool to room temperature. Beat 3/4 cup of whipping cream until soft peaks form. Fold the whipped cream into the cooled chocolate mixture. Stir in 1/2 cup of the finely chopped hazelnuts. Chill 30 minutes.

Beat remaining 2 cups of whipping cream until soft peaks form, then fold in the remaining 1/2 cup of chopped hazelnuts. Chill until ready to frost cake.

Place 1 cake layer on cake plate. Spread 1/2 of the chilled chocolate mixture over top. Add another cake layer. Spread with other 1/2 of chocolate mixture. Top with last cake layer. Frost entire cake with hazelnut-whipped cream. Place 12 whole hazelnuts around top outer edge of cake as a garnish. This cake should be kept in the refrigerator.

Nutrition

201 calories; protein 2.5g; carbohydrates 18.4g; fat 13.9g; cholesterol 30mg; sodium 157.3mg.

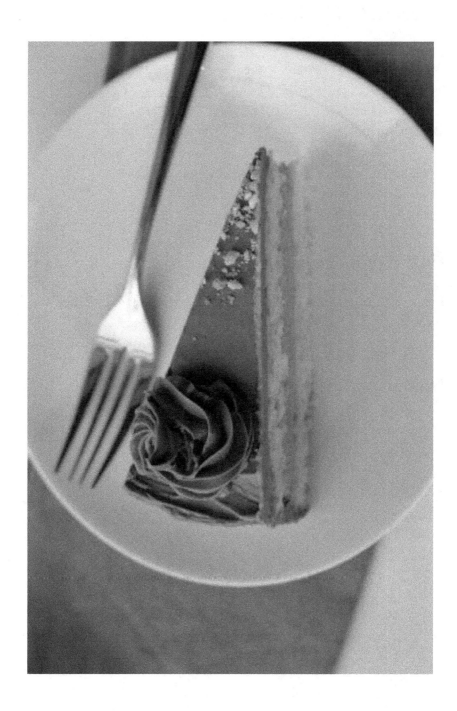

Coconut Coffee Mousse

Prep:10 mins
Additional:3 hrs 50 mins
Servings:8

Ingredients

1 (8 ounce) container frozen whipped topping, thawed
¼ cup flaked coconut
2 tablespoons coffee flavored liqueur

Directions

Fold coffee liqueur and coconut into whipped topping until well combined. Pour into 8x8 inch baking dish and freeze 4 hours, until firm.

Nutrition

110 calories; protein 0.2g; carbohydrates 8.3g; fat 6.6g; sodium 1.4mg.

Pumpkin Ice Cream

Prep:15 mins
Cook:15 mins
Additional:3 hrs
Servings:8

Ingredients

1 ½ cups half-and-half
¾ cup white sugar
½ teaspoon vanilla extract
1 ½ cups canned pumpkin
¾ teaspoon pumpkin pie spice
6 egg yolks
1 ½ cups heavy whipping cream

Directions

Heat half-and-half in a saucepan over medium-low heat to just below a boil, about 5 minutes.
Beat egg yolks, sugar, and vanilla extract together in a bowl using a whisk until smooth. Gradually pour half-and-half into egg mixture to temper the eggs; add pumpkin pie spice.
Pour the half-and-half mixture back into the saucepan; cook and stir over medium-low heat to just before boiling until mixture thickens, about 10 minutes. Remove saucepan from heat and beat pumpkin and whipping cream into half-and-half mixture until smooth; strain through a fine-mesh strainer into a bowl. Refrigerate pumpkin mixture until completely chilled, at least 1 hour.
Transfer pumpkin mixture to an ice cream maker and follow manufacturers' Directions for making ice cream.

Nutrition

342 calories; protein 4.7g; carbohydrates 26.3g; fat 25.2g; cholesterol 231.6mg; sodium 152.4mg.

Sugar Cookies

Servings:24

Ingredients

1 ¼ cups white sugar
½ teaspoon cream of tartar
1 cup butter
3 egg yolks
2 ½ cups all-purpose flour
1 teaspoon baking soda
1 teaspoon vanilla extract

Directions

Preheat oven to 350 degrees F. Lightly grease 2 cookie sheets.
Cream together sugar and butter. Beat in egg yolks and vanilla.
Add flour, baking soda, and cream of tartar. Stir.
Form dough into walnut size balls and place 2 inches apart on cookie
sheet. Don't flatten. Bake 10 to 11 minutes, until tops are cracked and
just turning color.

Nutrition

163 calories; protein 1.8g; carbohydrates 20.5g; fat 8.4g; cholesterol
45.9mg; sodium 108.2mg

Fruit Trifle

Prep:15 mins
Additional:1 hr
Servings:12

Ingredients

1 (12 ounce) package frozen blueberries
2 (16 ounce) tubs reduced-fat frozen whipped topping, thawed
2 cups chopped fresh strawberries
1 (12 ounce) package frozen peach slices, chopped
1 (6 ounce) container fresh raspberries
1 prepared angel food cake, cut into chunks

Directions

Pour the blueberries into a strainer, rinse with water, and shake off
excess water. Spread the berries out onto paper towels to dry slightly.
In a deep, clear glass bowl or trifle bowl, spread a layer of angel food
cake chunks. Scatter the cake with chopped strawberries in a thin layer.
Sprinkle the strawberries with a layer of blueberries, followed by a
layer of chopped peach slices. Sprinkle a few fresh raspberries over the
peaches. Dollop a layer of whipped topping, then repeat layers until all
cake and fruit has been used. Finish trifle with a layer of whipped
topping. Cover the trifle, and refrigerate until chilled, about 1 hour.

Nutrition

295 calories; protein 2.3g; carbohydrates 55.1g; fat 8.9g; sodium
212mg.

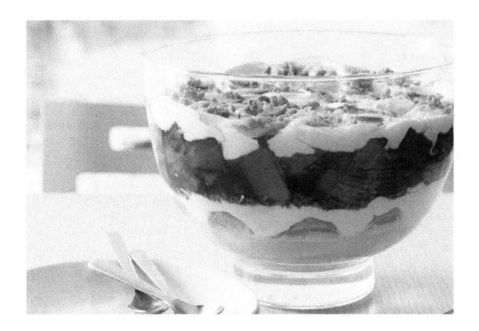

Blueberry Granita

Prep:

15 mins

Additional:

4 hrs

Total:

4 hrs 15 mins

Servings:

4

Yield:

4 servings

Ingredients

2 ½ cups blueberries

½ cup white sugar

¾ cup water

1 tablespoon fresh lemon juice

Directions

1

Blend the blueberries and sugar in a food processor until smooth; strain through a fine-mesh strainer, pressing with a wooden spoon to separate the blueberry puree from any chunks of skin or seeds.

2

Stir the strained blueberry puree, water, and lemon juice together in a shallow glass baking dish or tray. Place the dish in the freezer; scrape and stir the blueberry mixture with a fork once an hour until evenly frozen and icy, about 4 hours. Scrape to fluff and lighten the ice crystals; spoon into chilled glasses to serve.

Nutritions

Per Serving: 149 calories; protein 0.7g; carbohydrates 38.5g; fat 0.3g; sodium 2.3mg.

Lemon Cake

Prep:

20 mins

Cook:

45 mins

Additional:

1 hr 10 mins

Total:

2 hrs 15 mins

Servings:

12

Yield:

12 servings

Ingredients

10 tablespoons milk, divided

1 tablespoon dried lavender buds

1 ½ cups white sugar

½ cup butter, melted

5 eggs

¾ cup lemon juice, divided

1 ½ lemon, zested

2 cups cake flour

1 teaspoon baking powder

1 cup confectioners' sugar

Directions

1

Preheat oven to 325 degrees F (165 degrees C). Grease a fluted tube pan (such as Bundt®) generously.

2

Measure 5 tablespoons milk into a microwave-safe bowl. Heat in the microwave until warmed through, 30 to 45 seconds. Add lavender buds. Let steep to release their flavor, 10 to 15 minutes.

3

Whisk white sugar and butter together in a large bowl until creamy. Whisk in eggs, 1 at a time, whisking well after each addition. Add 1/2 cup lemon juice and lemon zest; mix until well-blended. Stir milk and lavender buds into the batter.

4

Sift cake flour and baking powder together in a bowl. Slowly fold into the batter, stirring well to prevent lumps. Pour into the greased tube pan.

5

Bake in the preheated oven until a toothpick inserted into the center of the cake comes out clean, 45 to 55 minutes. Cool in the pan for 5 minutes. Invert onto a wire rack to cool completely, at least 30 minutes.

6

Whisk remaining 5 tablespoons milk, 1/4 cup lemon juice, and confectioners' sugar together in a small bowl to make glaze; drizzle over the cooled cake. Let stand until glaze is set, about 30 minutes.

Nutritions
Per Serving: 329 calories; protein 4.8g; carbohydrates 56.3g; fat 10g; cholesterol 89.6mg; sodium 126.9mg.

CHAPTER 7: SMOOTHIES AND DRINKS

Dandelion Tea

PREP TIME 5 mins
COOK TIME 20 mins
TOTAL TIME 25 mins...
SERVINGS 4 cups...

INGREDIENTS

2 cup dandelion all parts
4 cups water boiled

DIRECTIONS

Clean dandelion
Boil water Pour boiling water over dandelion
Cover water and dandelions with a lid...

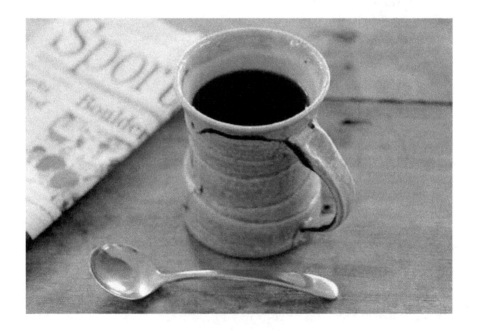

Lemon Pina Colada

YIELDMakes 2 servings

INGREDIENTS

1/2 cup canned sweetened cream of coconut (such as Coco López)
6 tablespoons citrus-flavored rum
1/4 cup chilled whipping cream
6 tablespoons white rum
3 tablespoons fresh lemon juice
Grated lemon peel
Ground nutmeg
4 cups crushed ice
3/4 cup pineapple juice

Directions

Place first 6 ingredients in large blender. Add ice. Cover and blend until smooth. Pour into two 14-ounce glasses. Garnish with grated lemon peel and nutmeg.
Coconut Rim
Dip the rim of each glass in water, then press into a bowl of coarsely crushed toasted shredded coconut. To crush the coconut easily, rub it several times in the palm of your hand.

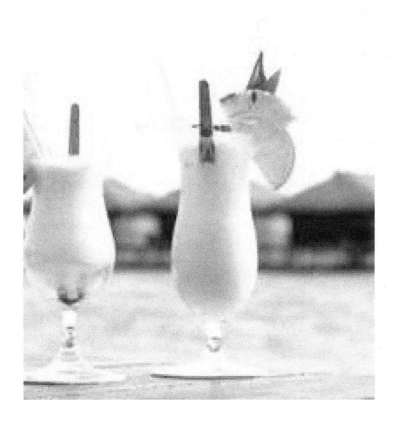

Ginger Tea

Prep:5 mins
Cook:10 mins
Additional:5 mins
Servings:1

Ingredients

8 ounces apple cider
1 (2 g) bag green tea
1 (2 inch) piece fresh ginger, peeled and sliced

Directions

Combine apple cider and ginger in a saucepan; bring to a boil. Boil for
2 to 3 minutes.
Place tea bag in a mug. Pour boiling cider into the mug, straining out
the ginger slices. Steep for 1 to 2 minutes. Remove tea bag.

Nutrition

133 calories; protein 0.2g; carbohydrates 33.1g; fat 0.1g; sodium
27.4mg.

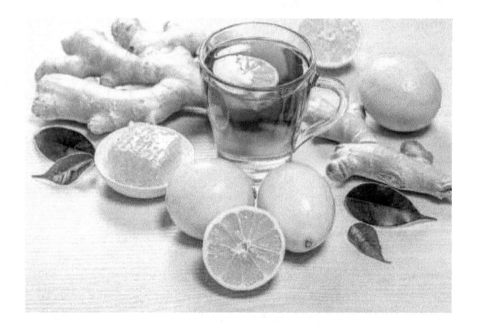

Beetrootroot ice

INGREDIENTS

ICE CREAM
200 g raw beetroot (about 2 medium beets – 100 ml freshly pressed beet juice)
300 ml (1 1/4 cup) heavy cream, 35-40% fat
finely grated zest from 1 lemon
2 tbsp. lemon juice
15 g fresh ginger
200 ml (3/4 cup + 1 1/2 tbsp.) milk, 3% fat
90 g (1/3 cup + 1 1/2 tbsp.) granulated sugar
1 tbsp. cornstarch
pinch of salt
1 tbsp. vodka (can be omitted)

DIRECTIONS

BEETROOT & GINGER ICE CREAM
Trim the edges of the beet roots. Peel them if they are very dirty, if not, washing them is enough. Cut them in smaller pieces and process them in a juicer together with the ginger. In a medium bowl, combine the beet juice, cream, lemon zest and juice.
In a small bowl, whisk together the cornstarch with 2 tbsp. of the milk. Heat the remaining milk, sugar and salt in a small saucepan until it comes almost to a boil and the sugar melts. Whisk in the cornstarch slurry and cook over low heat, stirring vigorously, until mixture thickens. Remove from the heat and mix with the beet juice and cream mixture. Stir until combined.
Let mixture cool completely. If you wish to speed things up a little, put the bowl in an ice bath and stir until cool. Cover the bowl with a lid or

plastic wrap and store in fridge until completely cold, preferably overnight.

Stir in vodka if using. Churn the ice cream in an ice cream maker according to your manufacturer's Directions.

Transfer ice cream to a freezer container. Smooth the top with a spatula, then loosely cover the surface of the ice cream with wax paper and freeze until almost solid, about 2-4 hours.

Conclusion

Kidney disease is now ranked as the 18th deadliest disease in the world. In the United States alone, it is estimated that more than 600,000 Americans have kidney failure.

These statistics are concerning, so it is essential that you take proper care of your kidneys, starting with a kidney-friendly diet.

In this e-book, you will learn that management creates healthy, tasty, and kidney-friendly dishes.

These recipes are ideal whether you have been diagnosed with a kidney problem or want to avoid it.

When it comes to your well-being and health, it's a good idea to visit your doctor as often as possible to make sure you don't experience problems that you may not have. The kidneys are your body's channel for toxins (like the liver), cleaning the blood of distant substances and toxins that are flushed out by things like food preservatives and other toxins.

Where you eat fluffy and fill your body with toxins, whether from food, beverages (for example, drink or alcohol) or even the air you breathe (free radicals are in the sun and move through your skin, through dirty air), and many food sources contain them). Your body will generally convert a lot of things that appear to be benign until your body organs convert them to things like formaldehyde due to the synthetic response and metamorphic phase.

An example is a large part of these dietary sugars that are used in sodas. For example, aspartame is converted to formaldehyde in the body. These toxins must be removed, or they can cause disease, kidney failure, malignancy, and various other painful problems.

This is not a situation that happens without any predictions; it is a dynamic problem and in the sense that it can be found as soon as it can be treated, change the diet, and it is possible what is causing the problem. You may still have partial kidney failure, as a rule. It takes a little time (or a completely terrible diet for a short period of time) to reach complete kidney failure. You would rather not have total kidney failure as this will require standard dialysis treatments to save your life.

Dialysis treatments explicitly cleanse the blood of wastes and toxins in the blood using a machine, taking into account the fact that your body can no longer be held responsible. Without treatment, you could die a very painful death. Kidney failure can be a consequence of long-term diabetes, hypertension, and unreliable diet, and can be the result of other health problems.

A kidney diet is related to the orientation of protein and phosphorus intake in your eating routine. It is also important to limit your sodium intake. By controlling these two variables, you can control the vast majority of toxins/wastes produced by your body and thus allow your kidney to function at 100%. If you do this early enough and really moderate your diets with extreme caution, you could prevent complete kidney failure. If you receive it early, you can fix it completely.

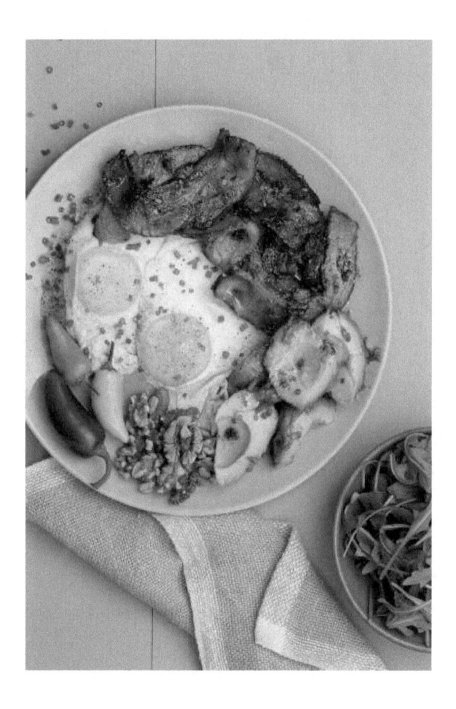

CPSIA information can be obtained
at www.ICGtesting.com
Printed in the USA
BVHW041722090621
609091BV00016B/2551